I0843302

Conditioning 201

JEWEL SWEENEY

Copyright © 2018 Jewel Sweeney

All rights reserved.

ISBN:1727024990

ISBN-13: 978-1727024999

DEDICATION

To the ladies of Sweeney Fitness that have come out week after week wondering what each night would hold, you made this happen! You keep me thinking of new ways to kick your butts and have fun with it; or at least "Jewel Fun."

Conditioning 201 is designed for classes of all sizes. When using these workouts with larger groups, check for enough equipment and plenty of space. Keep in mind the levels of all participants. Adjust any exercises or time frames for the class. These are fun workouts that will encourage participants to get moving and keep working towards their goals.

For any further explanations on exercises or workouts, contact Jewel Sweeney @ Facebook.com/SweeneyFitness

<u>Learning the Ropes</u>

 Inside and outside space is best. Make adjustments as necessary. Go through each group from A-E and repeat. Give 1-2 minute rests depending on your class needs.

Group A: 1 minute each.

1. Shuffle – about 5 yards distance
2. Jump Rope- if a person cannot jump the rope, they can jump in place
3. Foot Fire
4. Squat Jumps

Group B: Ladders: Running through each ladder and jogging back around. Total of 5 minutes.

1- Doubles- 2 feet running through each box
2- Singles – 1 foot in each box
3- Laterals – 2 feet in each box running laterally
4- Laterals second side
5- Jumping Jacks

Group C: 1 minute each. People rotate through stations.

1- Push Ups
2- Lunges
3- Plank
4- Dips

Group D: 5 minutes total

1- ¼ mile split

2- Rest

3- ¼ mile split

4- Rest

Group E: 1 minute each. People can rotate through or class can do it all at the same time.

1- Plank walks or Mountain Climbers- adjust according to class members
2- Ball Pass – use an exercise ball and pass the ball from hands to feet and back while laying on the floor. Arms and legs should open and close together.
3- High Knees
4- Crunches

Agility Rules

Inside and outside space is best. Make adjustments as necessary. Repeat each group before moving on to the next one. Give 1-2 minute rests depending on your class needs.

Group A: 1 minute each.

1- T- Runs – this is a typical athletic drill. Different sports may approach the same conceptual drill in slightly different ways. Choose which you feel is best for your group.
2- Obstacle Jump – Laterally jump over an obstacle. Choose an obstacle based upon your group. Banana hurdles are great, but if your group cannot jump high enough consistently, you can choose your own item, like a stack of cones.
3- Line Runs – quick feet over and back over a line drawn in the area.
4- Bounding – two footed long jump, as far as possible.
5- High Knees Up & Out – Drive the knee up like a high knee or an A-skip, lightly tap the foot down and bring it back up to the side. Switch sides. This is a high paced run/skip exercise.

Group B: Alleys – choose a 20 meter area to perform these exercises down and back for 1 minute each.

1- High Knees
2- Grape Vines
3- Butt Kicks
4- Power Skips
5- Sprint

Group C: Strength

1- Bear Crawl
2- Single Arm press
3- Leg Lifts
4- Side Lunge Kick
5- Sit Ups

Group D:

1- Plank Jacks
2- Driving Knees – pretend you are in a kickboxing class and bring an "attacker's" face to the knee.
3- Crossover Step
4- Punches
5- Jog

Boot Camp

I own a small truck tire that is about 55lbs and a larger tractor tire about 115 lbs. My sand bags are between 10-15 lbs. You can use what you have, or use this as an excuse to invest in more equipment! We do this workout at a local open field that has a ¼ mile track around it. It could be done inside, but it might get a little messy.

1- Small tire dead lift carry 30 yds
2- Sand bag toss 10 yds
3- Large tire flip 40 yds
4- Sand bag carry 20 yds
5- ¼ jog

Repeat through the system as many rounds as possible.

Walk Around the Block

We do the first part through a neighborhood. This could be done around a track or even in a gym (though less enjoyable).

Walk with extras : 30 minutes

- 2 min jog/ 1 min "extra"
- 2 min walk/ 1 min "extra"
- Extras can include, but are not limited to: walking lunges, walking squats, push ups, table top dips, high knees, butt kicks, skips, grapevines, shuffles, sprints, step runners on a curb, single leg squats on a curb, calf raises on a curb, box jumps on a curb, walking side lunges, inchworms, bear crawls, etc.

Inside: with partners – 1 minute each. Repeat 1-6.

1- Ball Pass push ups- use a small med ball. Do a push up with one hand on the ball. Roll the ball to your partner across from you. They do a push up with the ball and roll it back. Repeat with opposite hand on ball.
2- Tuck Jumps
3- Curve Up
4- Walking Push Up High 5's – Do a push up. Give your partner a high five. Walk to the side in push up form. Do a push up. Give your partner a high five with the other arm.
5- Flat Frogs – crouch in frog position, hands flat on the floor. Jump, kicking your feet straight out behind you with your hands stationary. Let your body rest on the floor. Push your body up and jump the feet back to the hands.

6- Partner Rotation with Ball – stand back to back with a medicine ball. Rotate and hand the ball off to your partner. Rotate back to the other side to get the ball. Change directions during second set.

Double Fun

Group A: 1 minute each. 2 min break after first 12 mins. Each person will stay at the station for two minutes total. They will perform the (a) and (b) exercises listed at the station. Then they will rotate to the next station.

1a- Box crosses

1b- Box Runners

2a- Bound / Back peddle

2b- Plank Jumps side

3a- Tire flip (55 lb tire) – use about 20 meters of space

3b- Tire pull (55 lb tire)

4a- Skaters

4b- Single leg hop over

5a- Shuffle – use about 20 meters of space

5b- Grapevines

6a- Trampoline Hop

6b- Trampoline Run

Group B: 1 min each – rotate through each of the six items. Repeat. Give 2 minute rest.

1- Lat Pull Downs
2- 6 inches
3- Squats
4- Plank with Moving Knees easy/med/hard
5- Superman
6- Knee Taps

Group C: finish the session until cool down and stretching.

¼ mile sprints – how many can you get in?

So Nice, Do it Twice

This workout begins in a similar format as the workout before.

Group A: 1 min each. 2 sets, 1 min rest between

1a- ladders back and forth – do runs and jumps from one end of the ladder to the other.

1b- ladders to stop sign – do runs through the ladder and sprint out 20 meters. Jog back and go again.

2a- butt kicks

2b- butt kick jumps

3a- box jumps

3b- step offs

4a- high knees

4b- hydra skip

5a- lunges with back peddle

5b- 180's/ 360's – jump turning 180 degrees 2, then 360 degrees

6a- Sumo to squat jumps

6b- touch downs

Group B: 1 min each, rotate through each exercise. Do 1 min Jumping jacks between every 2 exercises. Give 1 min rest between sets.

1- Step back press – using a band under one foot, do a reverse lunge and press up
2- Diamond crunch
3- Squat hold
4- Boat hold

5- Table top march

6- Crow push ups

Pre-Season

Group A: 5 mins continuous clock. In a 20-30m area marked off:

1- Jog back and forth

2- High knees/ Jog

3- Butt Kicks / Jog

4- Sprint / Walk

Group B: 1 min each

1- Ladders: Bunny hop, single leg hop, Jumping jacks

2- Shuffle cones – approx 10 yds apart

3- Zig zag cones – six cones about a meter apart in a zig zag. Push off and single let bound through the cones, then back peddle back to the start.

4- Foot fire

5- Jump rope

Group C: 1 min each

1- Push ups

2- Russian twists

3- Squats

4- Leg lifts

5- Table top dips

Love Potion No. 9?

4 groups 9 minutes each followed by inside workout.

Group A: Repeat 1 minute each for three rounds.

1- Walking lunges

2- Walking squats

3- Walking side lunges

Group B: continuing clock for 9 minutes

1- Large tire flip approx 30 yards. Large tire (115 pounds)

2- Jog back and to tire

3- Flip back

4- Tire burpees

Group C: Repeat 1 minute each for 3 rounds

1- Tire hits – small tire (55 lbs)

2- Run throughs

3- Runners

Group D: Repeat 1 minute each for 3 rounds.

1- Walking push ups

2- Shoulder holds

3- Table top march

Inside – 2 rounds

1- Ball crunch series- ball crunches 1 minute, oblique crunch on ball 1 minute, reaches on ball 1 minute

2- Ball plank – 1 minute

3- Ball pulls – feet on ball, hands in plank. Roll ball in and out 1 minute

<u>Fight Time</u>

Boxing: 3 minute rounds

- Box

- Sit ups
- Jump rope
- Box push ups
- Line runs
- Box
- Squats
- Jump rope
- Box
- Russian twist
- Line runs
- Box dips
- Jump rope
- Box
- Lunges
- Line runs

Repeat

<u>Deal With It</u>

Card Game – Each person picks 5 cards. Follow rules. Do each hand one at a time. Repeat as many hands as playable.

Ace- Burpees

2- Squats

3- Tuck Jumps

4- Sit ups

5- Diamond Push ups

6- side raises

7- Push ups

8- High knees

9- Cinderellas

10- Pistol squats

J- Jumping Jacks

Q- High Knees

K- Plank with knee kicks out

Joker- ¼ mile sprint

Hearts- 10 reps

Diamonds- 20 reps

Spade- 1 min

Club- Until the end of current song

Captain's Roll

Leadership Building: "Captain" rolls the di 5 times. While they do their exercises in three sets, they must pick an exercise from "Team Support" list for the team members to do through the entire set. Captains change after each round. Team only does 3 exercises, one time each set of the captain's workout.

Captain's Roll	Team Support
1- Squats	1- Butt kicks
2- Push Ups	2- Plank
3- Single Arm Press	3- A Skip
4- Chin Ups	4- V- Ups
5- Hand Stand Push Ups	5- Plank Jacks
6- Superman	6- Punch Crunch

7- Bench High Knees

8- Flutter kicks

9- Washing Machine

10- Toe touches

Try Outs

Go through each group once, then repeat.

Group A: Courtside 1 min each

1- Side line jumps
2- Foot fire
3- Shuffles – 6 ft distance
4- Foot fire
5- Mikan drill – lay up style (basketball). Step off one foot and drive the opposite knee up. Land crossing over towards the other foot, step off and repeat.

Group B: Field 1 min each

1- Ball slams

2- Ball taps

3- Toe taps – Opposite hand to foot, kicking up with a hop.

4- Ball taps

5- Jumping jacks

Group C: Core 1 min each

1- Plank knees to side

2- Negative crunch

3- Leg lift pop

4- Oblique crunch

5- Bat swing – slow, using a dumbbell

Group D: Strength 1 min each

1- Lunge and twist – use medicine ball or dumbbell

2- Hot potato toss – use medicine ball

3- Squat hold with bounce – 4 quick squats, hold the 5th for 5 seconds

4- Shared ball hold – partners hold the ball at shoulder length between them. Make harder by having people in a circle and each hand sharing a different ball with a different person.

5- Mule kicks – opposite arms and legs.

Repeat all!

<u>Rotate</u>

Group A: 1 min each, repeat. Have stations set up.

1- Jog – can be in place or a set distance

2- Push ups

3- Tuck jumps

4- Reverse lunge

5- Russian twists

Group B: 1 min each, repeat

1- High knees

2- Alternating planks

3- Plank jacks

4- Calf raise squat

5- Standing knee crunch

Group C: 1 min each repeat

1- Butt kicks

2- Table top

3- Lunge jumps

4- Duck walks

5- Big flutters

Group D: 1 min each, repeat

1- Washing machine

2- Inch worms

3- Long runs

4- Step ups

5-   Boat hold

In It Together

Do groups A-C then repeat at the end. Do 3 rounds.

Group A: 5 mins. Going down and back together approximately 30 yds. All who finish before the last person do jumping jacks or running in place. Once the last person is back, everyone starts the next move.

- Jog down//jog back
- High knees//butt kicks
- Shuffle//shuffle
- Skip//back peddle
- Sprint//jog

Group B: 1 min each. Rotate each person through station.

1-   Flip large tire to stop sign
2-   Pull small tire to stop sign
3-   Ladders – run series
4-   Ladders- jump series
5-   Walking squats

Group C: 1 min each. Rotate each person through station.

1- Jump rope

2- T-runs

3- Cone over runs

4- Squat jumps

5- Box steps- running if possible

How Many Can You Do?

How many sets can you do? Do each group by letting participants rotate through the exercises as they choose. Nobody waits for anyone else on exercises, but stays within the groups together.

Group A: 5 mins. 1 min rest. Repeat.

1- Lat Pull downs x 10-15

2- Box jumps 30 secs

3- Kettle bell swings 10-15

4- Curve Up 30 secs

5- Bridge and fly with band 10-15

Group B: 5 mins. 1 min rest. Repeat.

1- Wall sits x 30 secs

2- Sprinter kicks x 30 – Be in a "starting block" position. Kick the back leg up. Repeat on other side.

3- Lunge skips x 30 – Drop into a half lunge. Jump, kicking the back leg up driving the knee. Repeat on other side.

4- Ab Bicycles x 30

5- Band pulls apart x 10

Group C: 5 mins. 1 min rest. Repeat.

1- Skater touch x 20 – Step laterally keeping body bent like a speed skater. Touch opposite hand to floor, kicking back leg long.

2- Box cross x 30

3- Cleans x 10

4- Reaction ball x 10 catches

5- Ball crunch x 30

Group D: 5 mins. 1 min rest. Repeat.

1- Ab roll x 10

2- Skaters x 30 – full jumping

3- Single leg squat x 10

4- Cresent pose 30 secs

5- External reach x 10 – place weight in one hand and raise that arm to 90 degrees at shoulder and 90 degrees at elbow. Stretch the arm out in front to a toe touch with the opposite leg.

<u>RUN!</u>

Group A:

Run 1 mile

Group B: 10 minutes – Repeat as many rounds as possible in the 10 minutes.

1- Sandbag carry to line 30 yards away
2- 10 Jumping Jacks
3- Sandbag carry back
4- 10 jumping jacks
5- Pick and rotate each round- 50 Jump Rope, 15 Squat Jumps, 30 Runners, 10 Shuffles

Group C: 5 minutes – repeat as many rounds as possible in the 5 minutes.

1- Sand bag overhead lifts x 10
2- Push ups x 10
3- Sandbag sumo squats x 10
4- Lunges x 10 walking
5- Sledge hammers x 20

Repeat groups B & C as needed depending on the time of Group A.

<u>Divide and Conquer</u>

Each person goes to a different group. Have multiple of equipment for more than 5 people

Group A: Kettle Bell

-double arm, single arm, alternating, double arm

- sumo squat, high row, curl, tri extension

- side raises, bicycles, leg crawls

Group B: ladders 3 rounds. Run through the ladder and out about 20-30 yards. The first is the ladder activity, the second is how to get to the end point 30 yds away. Jog back to the start of the ladder each time.

- Doubles to skips
- Singles to sprint
- Lateral to shuffle
- Lateral to shuffle opposite side
- Skip one to sprint

Group C: Exercise ball.

- Push ups, hamstring curl, crunches, back ext, squat and press, marches, plank with feet on, rotations, Hip ab/adduction, ball pass

Group D: rower

-row 5 mins

Group E: Med ball

- Ball slide push ups, in knees bridges, negative crunch, ball slams, ball in knee back raise/ham and quad, ball in knees raises, chest pass bridge, ball in knee squats, ball to knee crunches

Tiresome Work

Group A: Stations – How many can you do? 1 min each. Repeat

1. Box Jumps
2. Tire flips
3. Cone over jumps
4. Push ups

Group B: 15 minutes – How many can you do?

¼ mile and self guided rest

Group C: 1 minute each. Repeat

1- Walking lunge
2- Walking squat
3- Bounding
4- Walking side lunge

Group D: 1 min each. Repeat

1- Dead lift tire carry + 10 tire burpees

2- Hand Stand push ups

3- Hammer curls

4- Superman

5- Squat jumps

6- Mountain climbers

50/50

Cardio – 25 minutes. Rotate through the groups as many times as possible.

- 50 box jumps

- 50 A skips

- 50 jump rope

- 50 box overs

- 50 B skips

- 50 high jumps

- 50 box crosses

- 50 sec sprint in place

Strength – 25 minutes. Rotate through the groups as many times as possible.

- 50 squats
- 50 push ups
- 50 pull ups
- 50 sit ups
- 50 lunges
- 50 second plank
- 50 bear walks
- 50 gator lunges

Recess

Group A-

Double ladder – using two ladders, place them next to each other. Each person will have four squares – 2x2. If you don't have ladders, you can draw four 1ft x 1ft squares.

For 20 minutes use the 4 squares for a variety of running and jumping activities. You can make them up according to the group. Have fun with it. Do each exercise for 45 seconds to 1 minute.

Examples: Running in and out left, right, left, right; Two foot jump in and out, skipping over the first two boxes or using them; bunny hop in an 'x' format; run past the first two front and back; or lateral jumps over the ladder spaces.

Group B: Next round- seated group ball pass. Use one medicine ball for every 3 people. Sit in a circle with backs in towards each other. Pass the med balls in a circle for 1 minute. Change directions for a minute.

Group C: 10 minutes running time.

Rock – Paper – Scissors

Play the old game of rock paper scissors. Each loser must do 5 push ups. Everyone counts their wins. Each time a person wins 5 rounds, they run 30 meters and back. Continue for the entire 10 minutes

Group D: Repeat Group B

Group E: Repeat Group A. You can do the same routine you used to start the class or try a new set!

www.ingramcontent.com/pod-product-compliance
Lightning Source LLC
Chambersburg PA
CBHW081828250726
48657CB00011B/3526